Therapeutic Shiatsu Massage for the Beginner

By: Alice Charles

Therapeutic Shiatsu Massage for the Beginner

By: Alice Charles

Table of Contents

Introduction

Our bodies accumulate a lot of physical, emotional, and mental stress as we go through our daily lives. It could be a deadline to be met, a pile of homework to be done, or just too much housework to finish---this *"everyday" stuff* that we deal with can make us want to pack up and leave even just for a few days. However, as there are bills to be paid, work to be done, and goals to be achieved, it's hard to just leave everything behind and take a break.

It is difficult to take proper rest nowadays because of how busy our lives can be. Most times, even when we take some time off to relax and do nothing, we still end up thinking about the work we left on our desks and errands that we still have to do.

This makes our break ineffective.

Our daily lives can be so hectic that it may sometimes feel like we do not even have time to breathe anymore. There are so many things placed on our plates that we just want to drop it and get a new, empty one. It is tempting to do this but it is not easy and right. What we have to do is really give importance to our physical, mental and, emotional well-being.

Taking a break and sleeping are not enough anymore. As we tend to have a lot of things on our minds, we need something that would help us take our mind off of things that worry us. We need to have something that would not only make us physically leave our work rooms but also mentally and emotionally take a break from all the stress that we face.

This may sound silly and impossible but there really is something that will do these for us. It is not a robot-you that would do your work instead, though. You are still going to have to get back to your work after but at least, you get to experience real and authentic relaxation.

What I am talking about is massage therapy—Shiatsu, specifically.

In this book, you will learn about the wonders massage therapy/Shiatsu does to people. You will also learn about the different types of Shiatsu.

This book contains a variety of information that will give you knowledge about massage and Shiatsu. It has tips and warnings, too, that you can use for future reference.

Most importantly, you will find out about the advantages and disadvantages of Shiatsu. This will help you to completely understand Shiatsu as an alternative healing therapy.

Chapter 1- Massage in General

Massage is generally intended to reduce body aches and stress. It gives your mind and body time to rest. Getting a massage does wonder to people. It is like hitting two, or more, birds with one stone as receiving treatment can relieve chronic conditions such as high blood pressure, arthritis, fatigue, diabetes, back pain, infertility, and depression.

Receiving massage treatment can be considered as just leisure by many people but it is actually something that is beneficial to one's everyday life.

Working on a schedule is something everyone is familiar with and as hard as it can be sometimes, we just have to live with it. Office workers who sit on their decks facing their computers everyday often have their backs and necks really strained, housewives tend to get sore all over their bodies because of doing a lot of housework, and students may find it hard to concentrate in class due to their bodies being strained for having to sit almost the whole day.

Physical and mental stresses are two different things but both are complementary. Fortunately, these 2 can be relieved by massage therapy.

Massage therapy is basically the application of various techniques which may include rubbing, compressing, kneading, stroking, and tapping to aid in healing injured or tight muscle tissues, improving circulation, and reducing stress as a whole.

The effects of massage therapy are usually overlooked by people. Aside from the aforementioned benefits, massage therapy also promotes better sleep, improve concentration, and increase one's overall sense of well-being.

It involves putting pressure on the body with vibration. It can be done with or without mechanical aid. Massages target muscles, ligaments, joints, lymphatic vessels and other connective tissues.

Professionals usually perform massage therapies on a massage table or a mat. People who are not experts can do it on any steady surface like the floor or a bed.

Depending on the type of massage being received, the client may or may not be fully clothed.

History

Massage has been around for ages that its exact year of appearance cannot be pinpointed. The most celebrated and famous civilizations, however—Greek, Roman, Indian, and Chinese—are said to have taken a huge part in the development of massage. The earliest records were traced in China 4000 years ago, around 1800 B.C.

Massage was practiced to heal aliments acquired from manual labor and paralysis. In Egypt, signs of hand and foot therapy or now popularly called as Reflexology were found in hieroglyphics carved on pyramids. The use of oils and spices to add to the healing aspects of massage therapy started in India through Ayurveda. Julius Caesar is also said to have received massage treatment almost every day to alleviate nerve pains. Hippocrates, on the other hand, attested to the benefits of friction and rubbing to relieve joint and circulatory problems. He recommended physicians to learn how to do this in order to properly heal people.

This idea had been opposed by many people in Europe but the overall idea of "healing through rubbing" spread across the world. Other countries like Thailand, the Philippines, and Japan were able to create their own versions of this therapy.

Japan's one of the most popular types of massage—Shiatsu—is what this book is specifically about but we are not going to tackle it just yet, as it is also important to learn more about the whole aspect of massage.

Types of Massage

Massage therapy has been around for thousands of years. Nowadays, if you want or need to get a massage treatment, you may be faced with over 250 variations. These massages include manipulating, pressing, or rubbing the muscles and soft tissues with the use of hands and fingers.

Choosing the best treatment to get can be confusing so here are a few of the most common/popular ones:

Swedish Massage

Swedish massage or the "classic massage" is the type of massage therapy that is most commonly used around the world. Unlike most Asian-style massages that are based on Qi, this is based on the concepts of Physiology and Anatomy. This was founded by Per Henrik Ling who was a Swedish physiologist.

It starts by warming up the body with light strokes and kneading in circular movements before moving to deeper muscles. This type of massage is gentle and relaxing. It also helps in the removal of body toxins as the massage strokes used follow the body's blood circulation.

Swedish massage requires the skin to be lubricated with massage oil because of the various strokes applied to the body. Without massage oil, rubbing will not be as smooth as it should be and would also harm the client's skin.

When receiving this type of massage, one has to remove all his clothes to give the therapist proper access to the body parts needed to be massaged. However, some people who are not comfortable with this are allowed to keep at least their underwear.

If you are new to receiving massages, this is the best type to take as it is very simple and is most likely available anywhere you go.

Reflexology

Reflexology is basically a foot massage but based on Dr. William H Fitzgerald's Theory of Zone Therapy which dictates that certain parts of the body correspond to different points or areas of the foot, this is mostly used by people who want to target parts of their bodies that cannot be reached by *hands* such as the liver, lungs, stomach, etc. This type of massage is very relaxing and is said to promote better sleep.

This type of massage is not painful but there are parts of the feet that may feel sore or tender. These parts will be given more time by the reflexology expert to remove the pain. The hands are the tools mainly used in this massage. Applying pressure on different areas or points of the feet will affect other parts of the body and would help in relaxation.

Aside from the already mentioned benefits, people come to receive this massage to cure digestive disorders, fix hormonal imbalances, and heal sports injuries, back pains, and arthritis.

Aromatherapy

Aromatherapy is the type of massage that uses essential oils to help improve the physical, mental, and emotional well-being of a person. It uses oils extracted from leaves, roots, stems, flowers, barks and other parts of a plant to help in boosting one's physical and psychological health.

The aroma of essential oils stimulates the brain. Essential oils can also be absorbed by the skin so they can go through one's bloodstream and aid in the body's self-healing. People can choose among a variety of oils but usually, the masseuse will suggest and use oil/s that would address one's specific needs. This kind of massage is energizing, stress reducing and relaxing.

Sports Massage

Unlike most types of massage, sports massage is not focused on relaxation. Its aim is to treat or prevent injuries and help improve an athlete's performance. This, though, is not only just for professional athletes. Anyone who has a busy day to day life that involves light or rigorous physical activities can ask to receive this type of massage. This is similar to Swedish massage but instead of using long and slow invigorating strokes, sports massage uses faster strokes and stretches the body.

Sports massage can be done before or after a rigorous activity. It is designed to reduce fatigue, improve endurance and flexibility, prevent injuries, and prepare the body and mind to do its best performance.

Hot Stone Massage

Hot Stone massage is also like Swedish massage only that heated lava massage stones are placed on certain points of the body to loosen strained and tight muscles. The stones used for the massage are smooth and they are used by the therapist as an extension of their own hands or as a tool to give more concentrated pressure. The heat from the stone relaxes the client and helps warm up the stiff muscles so the practitioner will be able to work on the client's soft tissues easier.

The stones are left on the body for about 20 minutes before practitioners gently apply pressure to massage the body. This helps in relieving stress and reducing muscular tension.

Thai Massage

Thai massage is a combination of massage and stretching developed in Thailand. This was influenced by various traditional massage and medicine systems found in China, India, and Southeast Asia.

This was performed by Buddhist monks in the past as a part of Thailand's traditional medicine.

During the massage, the therapist will use his or her knees, hands, feet, and legs to reposition the client into a series of different yoga stretches.

This type of massage is done on the floor. Like in Shiatsu, the receiver need not remove some clothing and change into loose fitting garments to give ease-of-access, to undergo this massage. Oils and lotions are also not needed.

This type of massage uses stretches, compression, and light pressure to bring balance back in the body's system. It leaves the body energized and rejuvenated after the massage.

Shiatsu Massage

Shiatsu massage is an ancient form of healing used to cure different health conditions like nausea, vomiting, and headaches. It is also known to treat depression and anxiety.

Chapter 2- Shiatsu Massage

In the ancient times, it is believed that the human body is a great source of energy. This energy is called Qi. For the body to function well this Qi must follow the principles of Yin and Yang— it should be well-balanced. It is said that the imbalance of Qi is the root cause of body aches and many diseases, so Japan has the famous Shiatsu massage to help Qi flow through one's body to freely to maintain and promote good health.

QI and the Meridians

Qi is a primary concept of many traditional eastern medicines. It is often translated as "life essence," "life force," and "energy flow." Qi is described as the energy that nurtures and maintains the body, mind, and spirit. It flows along the body and changes rapidly. It can easily be replenished and reduced every day.

This concept came from the Chinese philosophy of Qi which means "breath." In Japanese, the word Qi can be associated with different words like spirit, heart, and mind. The word is often used in many ordinary everyday expressions about attitudes, characters, and moods. The word Qi is often distinguished as a word that means energy.

Qi flows around the body through the meridians. The energy goes around the areas where there is not enough Qi and drains off regions where there are too much. It regulates on its own and imbalances tend to get fixed on its own easily. However, if the blockage does not disappear and it starts to give a negative effect to the body, one is encouraged to receive Shiatsu to fix this.

Through a network of channels or lines, Qi is able to flow through the body. These invisible lines are called the meridians.

The principles of the Meridians are not only used in Shiatsu but also in many forms of oriental healing and medicine. Reflexology and Acupuncture are two of these.

There are 12 meridians in the human body. Shizuto Masunaga who was the founder of Zen Shiatsu developed this.

These meridians are mainly found in the head, lower back, arms and legs but some can be found in other areas of the body too. These meridians are said to be what connects the organs and the organs of the system in the body. Shiatsu helps energy reach these organs through the meridians.

The 12 meridians conceptualized by Shizuto Masunaga are as follows:

- Heart
- Large Intestines
- Stomach
- Small Intestines
- Spleen and Pancreas
- Lungs
- Liver
- Triple Heater
- Gall Bladder
- Heart Governor
- Kidney
- Bladder

Acu-Points

The concept of Acu-points is similar to acupressure and acupuncture points.

Acu-points are dots or tsubos found in the meridians. These points are similar to acupuncture and acupressure points.

These small dots are the parts which may possibly get blocked. Blockage in these areas can cause disturbance in the streaming of Qi.

There are traditionally 364 acu-points found in the 12 meridians of the body and 50 are often used in Shiatsu. Some who practice other types of Shiatsu may have more meridians and therefore more acu-points.

Besides the acupoints, there are also ashipoints which are the exact areas where Qi is blocked. The tsubos and ashis are used when diagnosing a patient. Signs of swelling, pain, and discoloration are used to know whether or not there is something wrong with the organ that the tsubos and ashis correspond .

History of Shiatsu

Shiatsu came from the words "shi" meaning finger and "atsu" meaning pressure. This is basically what this massage is all about—applying pressure to different parts of the body with the use of fingers and palms of the hands. Through squeezing and tapping of one's muscles, Qi will be able to flow properly and help the body heal itself from ailments.

Shiatsu massage was influenced by multiple healing arts. Historians say that it followed Chinese medicine practices as it is similar to Acupressure which, like Shiatsu, makes use of the fingers and palms to apply pressure to special parts of the body. Shiatsu, more specifically, is a mixture of Anma—a combination of Chinese acupressure and traditional Japanese massage, Do-In therapeutic massage, and Ampuku abdominal massage—a type of massage therapy usually received by pregnant women. Insights on physical therapy and anatomy from the West were also used in the development of Shiatsu.

Although Shiatsu has been around for a long time, it only gained its unique characteristic in the 20th century. Shiatsu originated from the Anma massage but as time passed, people realized that it only gave people relaxation and not much healing.

When practitioners realized the benefits of "finger pressure," they started calling their work "Shiatsu" to give more emphasis on its therapeutic benefits.

Shiatsu was once only practiced by the blind since it offered them livelihood and their sense of touch were considered especially apparent. However, as Shiatsu became more popular, more and more people, including the non-blind, started practicing it. And as

competition got tougher, people were forced to offer something new and different to their customers.
This is how schools of Shiatsu were born.

Types of Shiatsu

There are originally 2 schools of Shiatsu but as time passed, more and more types of it were introduced.

Nippon Style

This is the type of Shiatsu most often found in Japan. This style of Shiatsu was invented by Tokujiro Namikoshi. It is said that he was able to come up with this when his mother developed Rheumatoid Arthritis in her joints and there were no doctors in the town they lived in to heal her. As he always vaguely pressed on his mother's joints to help her ease her pain, he figured that stroking and pressing parts of the body that hurt could help lessen soreness.

Rather than energy channels, Nippon or Namikoshi style concentrates more on special points and the overall structure of the body and the nervous system.

In 1925, Tokujiro Namikoshi established the Shiatsu Institute of Therapy and when it gained recognition, he moved to Tokyo to open the Japanese Shiatsu Institute.

Zen Shiatsu

Zen Shiatsu was established by Shizuto Masunaga. He came from a family of Shiatsu practitioners but was more interested in Western psychology and Chinese medicine theories. He studied Psychology and later used his acquired knowledge when he decided to pursue Shiatsu as well.

Masunaga trained under Namikoshi before he started learning about the history of the healing art. He then reintroduced the roots of traditional Shiatsu by incorporating the Five Element Theory and energy meridians to his own style. Because he studied Psychology, he added the psychological, spiritual, and emotional aspects of man in the development of Zen Shiatsu.

Zen Shiatsu is focused on the meridians so it can be strong or gentle, depending on one's needs. Zen Shiatsu practitioners aim to have a deep connection with their clients to see change or progress in their bodies.
This type of Shiatsu is most probably the most common in the West.

Tsubo Therapy

Tsubo Therapy or Acupressure Shiatsu was introduced by Katsusuke Serizawa. He was a student of Shiatsu, Chinese medicine and physical therapy whose focus was to understand and know the scientific aspects of energy meridians. He specifically studied Tsubos, or acu-points. He wanted to be able to explain the benefits of Shiatsu in a way that will be accepted by those who are more inclined in modern science.

Tao Shiatsu

Tao Shiatsu was founded by Ryokyu Endo. The focus of this type of Shiatsu is the expansion of the theoretical and technical bases of previous styles of Shiatsu. It goes back to the 20 years of Shiatsu's clinical existence.

This type if Shiatsu tends not only to the receiver of the massage but also to the practitioner. Ryokyu Endo aimed to promote the well-being of the two by making his version of Shiatsu respond to their contemporary needs. He concentrated on developing a type of Shiatsu that would be able to adapt to the ever changing world—society and environment wise—so that it can stay and be used as an effective healing therapy even after a long time.

Endo did not go far beyond the roots of traditional Shiatsu but he introduced new ideas that made his version of Shiatsu revolutionary.

He introduced 24 meridians, instead of 12, and improved the manner of treatment and diagnosis.

Quantum Shiatsu

Quantum Shiatsu was influenced by Quantum Physics specifically by the Theory of Relativity. This is based on Pauline Sasaki's work which instead of focusing on the physical body, concentrated more on the energetic body.

This style of Shiatsu incorporates concepts from Quantum Physics that shows how the body can function as a growing and constricting field of vibrations.

Quantum Physics was used to regulate faster and more expansive energy in the body. Through this, Chakras and meridians were included to Shiatsu's principles as a form of healing art.

It creates an integrated and fit environment for spiritual and physical healing and development to happen. It helps the energetic body to function consistently.

Ohashiatsu

Oha Shiatsu is one of the most unique types of Shiatsu. It is about having a true physical, spiritual, and psychological harmony between the practitioner, or the giver, and the client, or the receiver.

Its focus is on synergism and communication and the self-development of the two.

It uses limb rotation, touch techniques, and stretches in a flawless stream of movement. It improves movement, endurance and flexibility, strengthens and enhances posture, revitalizes Qi and spirit, and helps one understand self, others, and the nature.

This was created by Wataru Ohashi.

Jin Shi Do

Jin Shin Do was founded by Iona Marsaa Teeguarden who was a psychotherapist by profession. She combined simple massage techniques and light yet deep finger pressure on the acu-points of the body to aid in the release of emotional and physical tension.

This type of Shiatsu lets the receiver get in touch with there feelings or emotions related to the condition of his body. This kind of approach to body and mind healing is a combination of Taoist yogic philosophy, Chinese acupuncture theory, traditional Japanese acupressure technique, Reichian segmental theory and breathing methods.

Barefoot or Macrobiotic Shiatsu

Barefoot Shiatsu was created by Shizuko Yamamoto. This type of Shiatsu is not only about the treatment alone, it promotes one's health and natural lifestyle even after the therapy.

Assessments are done to understand the recipient's way of living through the Five Transformation, and verbal, visual, and touch techniques. The recipient's pulses are also examined.

Barefoot Shiatsu uses gentle touch and pressure through different hand and barefoot techniques to help unblock the flow of Qi. It also aims to strengthen one's body and mind.

Macrobiotic Shiatsu gives receivers medicinal plant foods, corrective exercises, dietary guidance, tips on the right way of breathing, palm healing, Qi gong, and Self-Shiatsu.

Watsu

Watsu or Water Shiatsu started in 1980. Harold Dull learned Shiatsu in Japan and combined his knowledge on Zen Shiatsu's principles with his own ideas to develop a new kind of Shiatsu.

Warm water is used in practicing this massage because it puts people into very deep states of relaxation while they are awake. In this type of Shiatsu, the recipient is floating on water so there is no weight put into his vertebrae. This helps the practitioner move the spine in ways that cannot be done if the client were on land.

Watsu helps undo dysfunction on the pressure a rigid spine may have placed on the client's nerves by using slow and gentle pulls and twists on the body.

Chapter 3- Shiatsu Versus Western Massage

As mentioned earlier there are many kinds of massage all over the world. So why, of all these kinds, would you choose Shiatsu? How is it different from the massages that originated from the West?

Western massage and Shiatsu, despite having major differences, have similarities—both are designed to achieve relaxation, relieve stress, and promote good health.

Major Differences

Technique

Shiatsu, or Eastern massage in general, uses different techniques to soothe particular parts of the body. It focuses on energy meridian points that would give healing effects to various parts of the body.

Rocking, striking, pressure, and rolling are used instead of the general techniques of stroking and rubbing. Because of this, lotions and oils are not needed and the client can receive the massage fully clothed. This is the exact opposite in Western massage.

Western Massage includes deep tissue massage, soft tissue massage, sports massage, trigger point therapy, and myofascial release. Gliding, vibration, kneading, friction, and tapping are the major techniques used in Western massage.

Diagnosis/Approach

In Shiatsu, the practitioner gives diagnosis by observing the receiver. He must detect imbalances by examining the receiver's pulse. Finding the cause of the complaint is more important than treating the symptoms. Once found, the practitioner addresses the complaint through finger pressure and thus, would also relieve the client's body aches and pains.

Shiatsu brings stability back to the nervous system and stimulates the response of chemicals in the body to promote healing on its own. There are between 600 to 2000 points in the body that can be pressed and the therapist will put in a variety of pressure depending on the body part or pressure point.

If the muscles are tight, light pressure is applied to prevent the feeling of pain but as the muscles loosen, the pressure applied becomes deeper. By doing this, the body is able to release hormones and chemicals that will trigger the body's healing system.

In Western massage, the problem is directly addressed. The practitioner addresses the complaint and then considers the reason why it came up.

Unlike Shiatsu, which is considered a holistic kind of therapy, Western massage such as Swedish massage and Sports massage tend to focus on the areas of the body that hurt. Western massage practitioners do not always see the body as interconnected as well. In other words, western massage treats a specific area because it hurts. It does not consider emotional and mental causes.

Styles

Namikoshi Shiatsu is the official style used in Japan but over the years, more styles were created in Japan and other countries. However, even if there are new styles now, Shiatsu's main objective (treating the body by balancing Qi) is retained whether it is a kind that is traditional or modernized.

Western massage, on the other hand, can be divided into 2 groups—sports massage and well-being massage.

The goal of Sports massage is to help the recipient get in shape and ensure excellent performance while well-being massage aims to give the recipient a relaxing experience by creating a calm and peaceful ambience with the use of incense, music, candles, and colors.

In Sports massage, creating a tranquil ambience is unnecessary and almost always not given importance.

Chapter 4- Benefits of Shiatsu

It has been mentioned countless times that Shiatsu massage has a lot of benefits but in this chapter, we are going to be more specific about its benefits and effects on the body.

Shiatsu is designed to bring balance to the body's flow of energy. It does not only alleviate muscle pains, it also helps in curing a wide variety of ailments, disease, and symptoms.

Here are 5 benefits of Shiatsu:

Cures/relieves pain caused by Rheumatoid Arthritis and muscle stiffness

It was mentioned earlier than Tokujiro Namikoshi founded Shiatsu because he wanted to give her mom, who was suffering from Rheumatoid Arthritis, comfort. Today, Shiatsu is still used to relieve stiff and painful joints.

Rheumatoid Arthritis attacks the lining of joints because of inflammation of the body's tissues.

By applying finger pressure/Shiatsu to the hands and feet, symptoms caused by arthritis can be alleviated. Shiatsu can be very gentle so it is also safe to apply pressure direct to these painfully affected areas.

Shiatsu helps weak muscles and improves its overall health by improving the body's circulation. It can also relieve any type of muscle pain.

1. Pregnancy

Shiatsu is known to help women during monthly cycles to relieve menstrual cramps and anxiety but it is also very helpful to women who are going through pregnancy. It helps women who are in labor and can help the babies turn in the womb. Women who are overdue can ask for this massage to help induce labor. Morning sickness and swelling of the hands and feet caused by pregnancy can also by cured by Shiatsu.

2. Skin

Although this is not the number 1 reason why people ask for this massage, this is definitely one of its best effects—at least, in a woman's point of view.

Shiatsu massage helps enliven the capillaries of the soft tissues of the skin. It helps in keeping the skin smooth and moist by stimulating the sebaceous glands.

By receiving Shiatsu, skin will be resilient and safe from wrinkling and with the blood circulation improved by Shiatsu, the skin will be glowing.

3. Digestive and Circulatory System

Shiatsu massage helps improve circulatory and digestive system.

Through Shiatsu, one's cellular nutrition and circulation is improved. Shiatsu also helps the body digest food easily and eliminate waste products. It allows the body to store energy reserves which results to stamina increase. The body's metabolism and fat removal is also triggered by Shiatsu.

4. Headaches/Migraines

Migraine is an acute, painful headache that can last for a few hours to a few days. It often comes with sensory warning signs like flashes of light, tingling of arms and legs, nausea, blind spots, and increased sensitivity to sound and light.

Enlargement of blood vessel and the discharge of chemicals from nerve fibers loop around these blood vessels cause migraine headaches. A migraine headache decreases blood circulation and may cause people to feel even worse. There are some medications made to alleviate migraine but not all of them are effective.

As migraine is not something that one can easily get rid of, people ought to receive this type of massage because it helps the body relax. Shiatsu helps increase blood flow and circulation so it relieves stress and lessens the headache.

Aside from the 5 mentioned benefits, Shiatsu is also known to improve/prevent/help in:

1. Sleep disorders
2. Stroke recovery
3. Heart attack recovery
4. Chronic fatigue
5. Lymphoma
6. Sinusitis
7. Chronic bronchitis
8. Kinney disorders
9. Urinary Tract Infection (UTI)
10. Asthma

Chapter 5- Why Shiatsu?

We have already mentioned the many benefits of Shiatsu but if you are still not convinced, this chapter will tell you why it is best to choose Shiatsu among the other massages all over the world.

Shiatsu has no bad side effects

If you are taking pills or any type of medication to cure an ailment/s, you may suffer from side effects like headache, drowsiness, itchiness, etc. Although these are not especially severe, they can still be bothersome especially if you are just about to start your day.

With Shiatsu, these types of side effects never happen.

Alternative medicines and therapies are usually like this but because Shiatsu gives a lot of advantages, Shiatsu has become one of the most sought after alternative therapies.

Shiatsu is 100% natural

Again, alternative medicines and therapies are all natural but as the people of the society today favor maintaining overall health naturally, Shiatsu's 100% organic and holistic way of healing makes it very popular.

Shiatsu can be less pricey

One of the best benefits one can get from going for a Shiatsu massage therapy is its tendency to be cheaper in the long run. $100 may seem expensive for just one session but as Shiatsu has a lot of benefits, it may be better to have this kind of treatment rather than going to a hospital.

For example, if you have extreme muscle pains, going to a spa to receive Shiatsu therapy will only require you to pay once while going to a hospital to seek treatment would possibly require you to pay 5-10 times more. This may not even include the additional medications the doctor will ask you to take.

Shiatsu is relaxing and helps relieve pain

One of people's top reasons why they go for massages is because they want to relax and be relieved from body pains.

Like other types of massage, Shiatsu is done in a calm, peaceful, soothing, and quiet environment. Add to this the actual massage and the recipient is sure to feel relaxed, reenergized, and free from any kind of pain.

Shiatsu helps strengthen the body

Many medical experts may not agree with the capability of Shiatsu to prevent and cure diseases and ailments on its own but many patients have already supported the fact that it can.

Through Shiatsu's manner of manipulating the muscles of the whole body, the circulation of oxygen, lymph, and blood are improved and the body's immune system becomes stronger.

Chapter 6 - Techniques Used

A Shiatsu therapist uses a variety of techniques in order to perform the massage properly.

Pressure

Pressure is the primary technique used in Shiatsu. Any part of the body can be used to apply pressure but using the palm of your hand is the easiest. To do this, the practitioner has to do it very gently and without sudden movements. As the palms are spread on the part of the body (usually the client's back), the practitioner will have to breathe in and then lean forward and apply the weight over his hands as he breathes out.

The pressure must be applied slowly or gradually so that the recipient will feel relaxed and have enough time to say if the pressure being applied is too much.

It is best for the practitioner to move his weight rhythmically back and forth as he applies pressure. It is also important for him to imagine that he is breathing Qi into his client.

Breathing

When practicing Shiatsu, one must understand the importance of breathing. The practitioner's breathing has to be in tune with the client's.

Most practitioners do this by putting their hands on the back or abdomen of the client while matching his breaths with him before the actual session starts. This is done to make their Qi flow at the same time.

Kneading

Kneading or squeezing the body's soft tissue is helpful in getting rid of lactic acid and improving the body's circulation.

As we all know, helping someone loosen his tense shoulder by squeezing is effective. In using kneading as part of Shiatsu therapy, the practitioner and the client should work together in order for the client to get the amount of pressure he wants and could take to relieve his pain.

Kneading can be done by squeezing the fingers and thumb together or grabbing the flesh and squeezing it with the palm and fingers. This is helpful in stimulating Qi in deep tissues and just like every technique, it is best to do it rhythmically.

Stretching

The muscles produce lactic acid when used. If lactic acid stays in the muscle for a long time, the fibers will have a hard time sliding across each other and would cause the muscles to become shorter, stiff, and painful.

Through stretching in Shiatsu, the muscles will be allowed to return to their original state or full length. It is also a good method to free up the Qi that got stuck in the tight muscles.

This technique allows the body to release the stagnant Qi and the cramped emotions that go with it.

To do this right, the practitioner must do the stretches as slowly as he could and work with the client to know how much he can extend his muscles.

Manipulation

When people do not use or move their joints all the time, they can lose mobility and become stiff. Flexing these fully is part of a Shiatsu treatment.

To be successful in the manipulation of joints, the practitioner must first check the movement of the client's joints. Manipulating the joints must be done gently and the practitioner must not apply unneeded pressure to avoid injuries.

Palm Healing

Palm healing is similar to Reiki as both use the palms to give attention to body parts that hurt. In doing this, the practitioner should coordinate his breathing with the client's and as he breathes out, he must imagine that he is also sending Qi to his client.

Pounding

Pounding a client's body activates the Qi and helps improve blood circulation. It stimulates the body's surface and helps the client relax.

It is important to keep the wrists loose when doing this technique. The pressure must not come from the elbows and the hands must hit the body without inflicting too much pain on the client's body.

Tools in Practicing Shiatsu

Shiatsu is a natural way of healing the body. It does not require you to use anything else but your body. Different body parts give off different effects. To be able to do the techniques discussed, you must also know the right body part to use to project Qi and apply pressure.

Hands

Shiatsu means "finger pressure" so the hands are the most essential tools in giving the massage. The palms are used to apply even pressure on large areas of the body. The pressure applied through the hands can be easily regulated depending on the client's preference.

Thumbs

The thumbs of the hands are used in applying pressure needed to stimulate the body's acupressure points.

Elbows

The elbows are helpful in applying strong pressure on small areas of the body. If the practitioner or the client wants to concentrate on a specific spot, the elbow is the best body part to use as its sharpness gives off more powerful pressure.

Knees

The knees can also be used to apply strong pressure but unlike the elbows, the knees are used to spread pressure on a bigger or wider area of the body.

Feet

The feet, among all the other parts, are the simplest to use as it does not require much effort. The feet are used not only in Shiatsu as they can cover a wide area and can provide the right pressure. They are soft and flexible as well.

Chapter 7 - How to Do Shiatsu

To achieve relaxation, the ambience of the room where the therapy is going to take place must be calm and quiet.

Blinds, curtains, candles, and music are few of the things that could make a room's ambience placid. However, it all depends on the client's preference. If he would rather receive the massage without any music or candles lit up, then you should follow accordingly.

Shiatsu massages are usually done on futon mats but there are more and more spas that offer this treatment on a massage table. If you do not have a futon mat or a massage table, yoga mat will do. If you still do not have this, just make sure to make your client lie on a steady but comfortable surface.

Oils and lotions are not necessary when giving a Shiatsu massage. In fact, most practice this without using them. The client can receive the massage fully clothed but make sure that he wears light and soft clothing to allow easy movement.

If in case the client wants to have some kind of oil or lotion to be used on his skin as you work on him, do so. These induce therapeutic effects after all so it may add to the clients' mental and emotional healing.

When you have prepared all the things needed, you can now proceed to interviewing and diagnosing the client.

Interview/Diagnosis

The practitioner should talk to the client and know the condition of his health. He will examine the body of the client by checking the softness and hardness of the body to determine which parts should be focused on. The parts that are usually checked are neck, shoulders, the arms, legs, abdomen, and back.

Manipulation will be done throughout the body and the problem parts or areas will be given more focus.

An interview is important because it helps the practitioner understand the patient. Sometimes, the client knows exactly what to have healed but sometimes it could be the exact opposite. Having a short interview would make things easier for both the practitioner and the client.

Finding the Meridians

Because Shiatsu's main focus is the Qi and how it flows throughout the body, finding the Meridians of the body is one of the first things the practitioner does.

The practitioner would use his fingers to run through the spots where the meridians are usually are and feel for stiffness or tightness,.

Different types of techniques will be used to fix any irregularities found in the meridians. This will allow the Qi to flow through the body properly and would help loosen the knots in the muscles.

Other techniques can also be used to fix the problem areas. The intensity of the techniques used during the massage depends on the clients

Actual Massage

How the massage is going to be done depends on what the client needs—it can be done while lying down, kneeling on the floor, or sitting on a chair.

Where it is going to start also depends on the practitioner, too. Some practitioners prefer to start by massaging the neck and shoulders first before working his way down while some would rather start on the soles of the feet and work his way up.

If you want to try your hand at Shiatsu, here's a how to do it in 15 steps:

1. Start your practice on friends and family, it's seldom that anyone refuses a free massage. Ask the client to sit on a chair or kneel on the floor.
2. As you concentrate on the client's breathing, put your hands on his shoulders. Try to meditate and take subtle information about his emotional and physical condition. Using both hands, squeeze the shoulder muscles. Work from the neck to the ends of the shoulders. Do it rhythmically and knead until you and your client gets comfortable.
3. Place your forearms near the neck of the client and put weight on it as you lean forward. If the client wants more pressure, use your elbows.
4. Stretch the client's upper back by asking him to put his arms around your neck, and then lean back. Make sure to

support his back as you do this. Repeat when needed. This will help the shoulder become more relaxed

5. Pound on the shoulders.

6. Ask the client to lie on the floor. Kneel or stand beside him and then place palms on the upper back. Slowly put weight on your hands, pull back a little, and then go down.

7. Go back to the upper part of the client's back. Press your thumb near the spines. The distance must be a thumb width away. Put pressure on the thumb and go down once again. This part of the body follows the inner bladder meridian and doing this step activates many acupressure points.

8. Stand up and then put the ball of your foot on the client's buttocks. Rhythmically and firmly press your foot as you rock him from side to side to help the joints in his back loosen up. This may cause you to lose your balance so it's better if you can steady yourself by holding onto something while performing this.

9. Press your knee onto the back of the client's leg. Use the client's upper back or upper leg to support yourself. Move up to the client's upper leg but make sure not to put any pressure on the client's knee.

10. Kneel next to the client's leg and use your thumb to massage the calf muscles. As you work your way down, you will come across an acupressure point. This acupressure point is sensitive so ask the client to tell you the moment you press it.

11. Ask the client to point his toes toward each other. Massage the soles of the client by standing with your toes pointed away from each other. Stand on your toes and use your heels to apply pressure.

12. Work on the thighs of the client one by one by using your feet. After this, hold the ankles as you pick up the feet. Do

this until the knees are no longer on the ground. Swing the knees from side to side.

13. Hold onto the client's knees and lift them up to stretch the thighs and abdomen. Do this slowly and make sure that the client feels comfortable. If he starts feeling some kind of pain in his lower back, stop doing this stretch.

14. Put the knees back to its place on the ground and hold the balls of the feet and push them down slightly. This move stretches the back of the ankles. After doing this, pull your client's feet up to his buttocks. Communicate with him to get the most comfortable stretch.

15. To finish up, go back to rhythmically stretching the client's shoulders. This time, the shoulders will be much looser than when you started. After kneading and stretching the shoulder muscles. Pound on the client's back and buttocks.

Chapter 8- Tips and Warnings

TIPS

Before going through with a Shiatsu massage therapy, there are a few things both the practitioner and the client have to prepare.

- A few of these have already been mentioned like doing the interview, wearing loose and light clothing, and preparing a few things needed. Aside from these, the client and the practitioner must be in a calm state. Doing the massage requires the practitioner to breathe Qi onto the client. If the practitioner has negative feelings or is agitated while doing the therapy, the negative energy may possibly transfer to the client.
- It is ideal for the client to eat a few hours before the massage. If he is going to eat a heavy meal, he should do this at least 3-4 hours before the massage session.
- Consuming alcohol on the day of the massage is a huge no-no not only in Shiatsu but also in most, if not all, massage therapies.
- If the client is wearing any jewelry, the practitioner must make sure that he or she removes all of them.
- Perfume and aftershave are also unnecessary so it is better not to wear any.
- Just like the practitioner, the client must be in a calm state before the massage session. Although Shiatsu aims to relax the client, it is also good for him to relax on his own so his body would take the massage well. The same goes when the massage ends.
- The practitioner must let the client rest for 10-15 minutes after. A drink of water is also essential to help the body eliminate wastes.

Warnings

Shiatsu has countless benefits to the well-being of a person. One session is enough to see the difference it can make to the body.

So far, only the good stuff has been mentioned. So this time, let us talk about the disadvantages of Shiatsu.

This part of the book is not to discourage you to go through with the massage. This is only for you to be able to weigh the pros and cons of Shiatsu properly.

Everyone who is trying to sell something only mentions the advantages and uses of his product. Usually, people find out about the disadvantages later on and end up regretting buying the product.

Shiatsu can be the same for you so to help you see all the sides of Shiatsu, here are few things you have to keep in mind.

- One of the biggest problems people have with Shiatsu is its price. An hour or an hour and a half session would cost about $70.
  Unfortunately, if you want to receive a Shiatsu therapy to achieve healing and wellness and not just to relax, one session may not be enough.
- If you are the type of person who is not comfortable with having to be touched by a stranger or if you are new to having massages, receiving Shiatsu therapy may be troublesome for you.
  A part of the Shiatsu massage is pounding and/or stepping on the buttocks and upper thighs. Make sure that you are comfortable about this before going through the session because this step is essential to unblock the Qi's pathways

and asking to skip this may cause you to not get the full benefits of the massage.

- Shiatsu, for some people, can be quite long. A session takes about an hour to an hour and a half and it does not have the immediate effect a pain killer has. So if you are looking to quickly relieving your pain, Shiatsu is not for you.

- Also, some practitioners ask their clients to just breathe for 5-15 minutes to help there body relax and calm down. Some people find this unnecessary but it is important to follow through with this to be able to reap the benefits of Shiatsu.

- This massage therapy can cause muscle soreness and bruising if the practitioner pressed on the muscles too hard. This is more of the practitioner's fault rather than Shiatsu's, through. Many end up getting this side effect because they opt to get a "cheaper" therapy. Remember that even though it is not bad to receive massage from a new masseuse, it is still better to look for someone who has been doing it for a longer time to avoid these kinds of risks. SO IF YOU ARE JUST BEGINNING, GET LOTS OF PRACTICE. And take as many courses as you can find
Usually, people who are more experienced charge more. This brings us back to the first disadvantage mentioned—expenses.

Although Shiatsu has always been promoted as a "healing" therapy, there are still some diseases or illnesses that would do best without it.

All of the massage therapies all over the world have contraindications. Shiatsu is no different.

- People who have fractures in any part of their bodies, rashes, and open wounds should wait until they are completely healed to avoid complications.
- Receiving the massage when you have Psoriasis, fungal infection, varicosities, may find this is not ideal as it may irritate your skin more and make your condition worse.
- It is also only logical to not receive the massage when you have a contagious skin disease. Aside from doing so will cause your skin to break even more, it is highly possible for the practitioner to pick up the disease that you have. Do not put him in danger too.

The few mentioned so far are conditions that heal eventually so they can get the massage once they are well. However, there are a few more serious medical conditions that really prohibit people from taking Shiatsu.

- Experts say that people with any type of Cancer must avoid getting a Shiatsu massage. However, some practitioners of many massage therapies disagree and say that as long as the masseuse does not go near the tumor, it is okay to receive a massage.
  On the other hand, people who have Leukemia or other types of blood cancer are strictly not allowed to receive Shiatsu therapy. As Shiatsu improves the body's blood circulation, the cancer cell will spread faster.
- People who have severe nerve damage and Osteoporosis are advised not to have this massage as the practitioner may move sensitive points that would make their conditions worse.
- As mentioned earlier, one of the massages that influenced Shiatsu is the Ampuku abdominal massage. This helped Shiatsu become the type of massage that is safe for pregnant women. However, if a woman's pregnancy is delicate and at high risk, she

will not be allowed to undergo Shiatsu because this may cause bleeding or worse, miscarriage.

Chapter 9- Shiatsu: The Ultimate Stress Reliever

Stress is something everybody experiences—whether it be positive or negative. Although most believe that stress can only harm us, it actually has some good effects on people. Positive stress brings thrill to people's lives. It is the energy that pushes people to try doing things they do not usually have guts to do, such as making the first move, asking for a raise, or going bungee jumping.

People experience this kind of stress when they are faced with a demand that they can handle with confidence. People get this feeling when they encounter a situation where they want to put in effort to contribute something. It is that invisible push people get that makes them do something to achieve their goals. It is that thing inside of us that encourages us to take risks, to grow, to change, to adapt, and to fight.

Stress is an important part of our lives as the absence of it can cause people to lack motivation to fulfill their desire and hone their potentials.

However, stress can also have bad effects not only to our bodies but also to our minds.

Negative stress can cause people anxiety, fatigue, depression, and just plain unhappiness. It makes people feel miserable and make them feel like they will not be able to do anything right. People experience this kind of stress when a sudden change in their daily routines arise or when they encounter a situation that they think they cannot handle.

The feeling of unfamiliarity and discomfort can also cause this. As we can only choose where to work and not who to work with, we are often placed in a position where we have to forcefully adapt to our environment. Doing this is not easy for everyone and it is also not completely impossible to get into conflict with our colleagues. Although you may think that you do not care about not having good relationships with everybody at your workplace, the awkwardness between you and them can still unconsciously weigh on you and cause unwanted stress.

Add to this your boss, who you are sure is pushing you slowly (and surely) into a cliff, or rather beyond the capabilities of your once strong, now frail body, it can be such a nightmare!

One day, you may feel good about doing your job, but the next day, you just want to quit and hide in the comfort of your home's sofa.

This kind of feeling is common among people and despite this being normal, it should not be taken lightly. Stress can be short-term—it can intensify and disappear within a span of a few days, but it can also last for weeks, months, or even years.

The best way to get rid of stress is to develop a regular daily routine. You should take time to exercise and get your mind off of things for a while, start eating healthy, and try to develop a regular sleeping pattern. Correcting the imbalance stress has done to you is the best way to feel like you are in control again. However, as tempting as it sounds to get your life back on track, it is not really that easy to do. Just thinking about how and where exactly to start can already be quite stressful... and of course, we do not want that, do we?

So, what is the next best thing? It is taking time to relax.

Going on a vacation for a few days is a good idea but as busy as we are, we cannot just up and leave so taking an hour or two from our normal routine is more ideal as it will not take much of a toll on our busy schedules.

This is where relaxation through Shiatsu comes in.

Getting a Shiatsu massage treatment will not only be beneficial for the physical pains that you have. Throughout the book, I have said that this also helps in achieving relaxation a lot.

All of Shiatsu's healing effects may not be known by everyone but its capacity to bring someone into deep relaxation is very well-known and most of the time, the reason why people seek this type of massage.

Shiatsu is ideally done in a quiet and calm space but creating a room with a serene ambience is not really necessary. Although many spas and wellness centers use instruments like curtains, essential oils, and candles to create a certain type of mood, they are not really important in Shiatsu because the massage itself is what makes it very relaxing.

Shiatsu clears the blockages in the meridians and helps free your Qi so this makes you feel invigorated, revitalized, and revived, even, from your daily life. The techniques used and the 'human touch' add more to the rejuvenating effects of Shiatsu and may cause you to fall asleep. This helps release confined tension in your body.

Many massages are also capable of doing this but Shiatsu has something that makes people choose it over the others. Maybe it is how it releases tension and unblocks Qi at the same time or the fact that you can feel its effects just as the session starts. It is hard to give the exact reason as to why Shiatsu is very popular and is preferred by many people but those who have already tried this can confirm that it really does what it claims to do.

These days, we become so busy that we do not get to enjoy life. Taking time to receive a Shiatsu massage treatment will be the answer to this.

A Shiatsu massage session may only last for an hour or two but its effects on the physical, mental and emotional state of the body lasts for a long time. As it gives you time to relax and unwind, the body is able to free itself from all the stress that it has gathered over time. We may not notice it all the time but our bodies accumulate stress from the littlest things.

There are days when we are extremely irritable and do not feel like functioning at all. This is because our bodies are telling us to stop what we are doing and take time to wind down.

Taking a break once we have finished everything we are doing sounds like a great idea. However, we will never be able to completely empty our plates. We are just going to end up pushing our break back until we completely forget about it.

We have to remember that when the body is tired, we should give it some rest. If we cannot give it a day or two, then go for something that is quick, easy, and efficient.

Shiatsu is the ultimate stress reliever not only because it eases our body's aches and soreness but also because it is something that we can use to help heal our mind and body as a whole.

Think of Shiatsu not only as a means to relieve stress but also as a reward for always working so hard. Our bodies can only do much for us and it is only right for us to treat it well.

Chpater 10 - Becoming a Shiatsu Massage Specialist

Becoming a Shiatsu massage therapist is rewarding—not only in terms of monetary compensation but also its effect on one's well-being. A Shiatsu specialist's salary depends on his working arrangement but one can usually earn $100-200 dollars per session.

Learning Shiatsu is beneficial, not only for you, but for your friends, and family as well.

To become a Shiatsu practitioner, one has to learn how to do it properly. Undergoing training and obtaining certification is required to be able to practice Shiatsu professionally.

Learning Shiatsu

Someone who wants to become a Shiatsu therapist must have a natural passion for healing and interest in alternative medicine as enrolling in an institute would not only teach you how to do the massage—you will also learn about Anatomy and physiology of the human body.

You will learn about the pressure points, Meridians, and Tsubos that we have talked about throughout the book. Zen, Anma and Namikoshi Shiatsu will also be taught and you will be given a few important pointers about Chinese medicine.

Some institutes offering Shiatsu programs require you to take a course that lasts 300 to 700 hours. You can choose to study and specialize in different types of Shiatsu. Your load depends on what you can handle so the duration of the whole program may vary.

Training to become a masseuse can cost as much as six thousand to twelve thousand dollars. It is quite expensive but it already includes classroom work and hands on training and practicum so one is sure to learn and understand the essence of Shiatsu.

Shiatsu Training Institutes

If you really want to learn and become a licensed Shiatsu practitioner, then enrolling in a shiatsu institute will be very helpful.

Shiatsu has become a very popular massage therapy all over the world so it is not going to be hard to find a school that would help you become a specialist. Most schools or institutes have their own websites, if you cannot find the best school for you, going online and looking for schools would be advantageous.

www.ingramcontent.com/pod-product-compliance
Lightning Source LLC
Chambersburg PA
CBHW070623290526
45790CB00002B/972